BEAUTIFUL ME

ALL ABOUT HEALTHY LIVING

IRUOMA AWO

TABLE OF CONTENTS

Chapter 1 You need to know

Chapter 2 Be proud of and love yourself

Chapter 3 A lifestyle or a project

Chapter 4 Do it yourself (DIY)

Chapter 5 Meal suggestions

Chapter 6 Recipes and procedures

Chapter 7 Welcome on board

Other Books By Iruoma Awo

Chapter 1 You Need to Know

Until a problem is identified, the appropriate remedy cannot be administered. You need to know what it is you have been doing over time that has gradually led your body to its current state. It could include: activities you started or stopped doing, drinks you started or stopped drinking, foods you started or stopped eating, pills you started or stopped taking or an increase or decrease in your general consumption level. Till this milestone is covered, there is unfortunately no further headway that can be established.

How did I get here?

It is not out of place to see people being surprised about how much weight they have gained over time. They sincerely do not know how it happened. Hence, the need for them to be pointed to what it is they need to do better. Most of the time; such people live in denial of what it is they really eat. For instance:

- I eat healthy meals, yet I am this big.

6   Beautiful me; all about healthy living

- o Sure?

- ■ I never eat breakfast but I am still gaining weight.

  - o Skipping breakfast would result in over eating during the day. Unless you are fasting, please have your breakfast. What do you have for lunch and dinner?

- ■ I work out often but have lost no weight.

  - o How much calories do you burn while working out and how much calories do you consume after working out?

A CLOSER LOOK

A closer look through the magnifying glass; can you see the reflection of you in any of these?

1. Although you are satisfied, you still go for more food because the pot is not yet empty. The best thing to do is to pack up the remaining food and store in the deep freezer.

This would prevent you from getting tempted.

2. You have decided to enjoy your life. Your understanding about enjoying life is eating anything anyhow. You need to think again. You might end up cutting your life short and not enjoying it at all.

3. What do you have stored in your drawer at home and at work? What do you have stored in your hand bag?

4. How much alcohol do you consume? Alcohol has almost the same calorie content as pure fat, 7 calories per gram. 1 pint of alcohol equals 200 calories.

5. Do you hold on to that biscuit can or chocolate box until its content is empty?

The stated questions above embody calories that are easily over looked. Two of such instances are described below.

- You may not have breakfast but you nibble on those stored items in your drawer. Those may not be breakfast as you say, but that does not eradicate their calorie content. You consume them and the calories count, whether or not you recognize them as a meal.

- You have a meal with a glass of champagne. What is most of the time taken into consideration is the meal itself and not the glass of champagne. A glass of champagne contains 95 calories. If your meal contains 650 calories; it means you are totally consuming 745 calories at a sitting. Imagine how much calories you would be consuming when you have more than a glass of champagne.

It is advisable to cultivate a moderate drinking habit as alcohol has the potential of making weight loss difficult. You can occasionally give yourself a treat and this should be moderately done.

WHY DO YOU WANT TO ADD OR LOSE WEIGHT?

This is a question you need to ask and answer yourself. If you want to add or lose weight because of anyone else other than yourself, your action is not likely to be sustainable. You are your best motivator, not anyone else. Do it for you and not for any other person. When you have the desire to add or lose weight, this desire energizes you. It empowers you to be able to follow through actions, necessary to transport you to your desired destination. All you need to do is make it happen.

CHAPTER 2 BE PROUD OF AND LOVE YOURSELF

Being proud of and in love with yourself is the starting point for improvement. You may not like the way you look, but you need to uphold your pride because that is what you need to work out a change. Hold your head and shoulders high, being conscious of the fact that you are a work in progress. If you are ready for a change, you would encounter a change. But you will not encounter a change if you keep doing the same things the same way. On this path to healthy living, great efforts would be required and great sacrifices would need to be made.

EXERCISE

Exercise is about keeping your body in motion. It is a crucial complement to living a healthy life. It could involve going to the gym, running, home gymnastics, stairs climbing, walking, cycling, dancing, swimming or skipping. It boosts energy, increases heart and lungs efficiency and reduces the risk of stroke and heart attack. It increases the metabolic rate and makes it easier to maintain a healthy weight. It absorbs stress, keeps you flexible and leaves you refreshed and fit. If you have not been involved in any form of exercise before now, it is time to get started.

One of the ways to make exercise less boring is by forming an exercise group. A group consisting of individuals with whom you share the same goals. This helps you as well as the other group members stay motivated. When you begin to see results, you become even more motivated to continue and ready to go the extra mile.

CRAVINGS

Cravings have to do with the brain and hunger has to do with the stomach. Cravings are to be appeased and not suppressed. When you suppress your cravings, you are only preserving a radical consumption attitude for a future date. This means that there is a tendency of having less of that item which you have a desire for, if you appease your cravings and more of it, if you suppress your cravings.

Cravings could either be long term or short term. Long term cravings are consistent and they inform you about the state of your health. It notifies you of some deficiencies you may be having. For example, salt cravings indicate low levels of calcium, magnesium and zinc. A remedy for this is; frequent exercise, consumption of olives, tomatoes and leafy greens. Still reaching out for salty foods or snacks while at this remedy, may occur.

Short term cravings are not consistent and provide little or no information about the state of your health. For example, you get this feeling of wanting to eat chocolate. You walk up to the chocolate box you have at home; pick a piece of chocolate, have a bite and the craving is gone. You do not need to consume the entire piece of chocolate for the urge to disappear. You would realize that you do not return to that box of chocolate until after several months, although it is right there in your home.

Chapter 3 A lifestyle or a project

Dieting is sometimes indulged in, for the purpose of being able to fit into an outfit. An outfit carefully selected for a forthcoming high class societal occasion. After the occasion in question, there is an automatic reversal to what is termed "normal life". That is a project and not a life style. A project has a start time, end time and a goal to be achieved. Healthy living should neither be viewed nor implemented that way. Your life is priceless and should be handled with long rather than short term principles. Instead of dieting, try living healthy.

Healthy living

Living healthy can be as simple and interesting as you want it to be. Quit skipping meals. Food is to be eaten. Eat and do not starve yourself. Starvation is neither the pathway to weight loss nor healthy living. Here are some tips on how healthy living can be upheld as a lifestyle and not a project. These tips are able to keep you away from strenuous exercises, help you stay healthy and restrain your waist line from enlarging. As the routine is incorporated, your body gets adapted to it with time.

Watch **how (quantity)** you eat, **what (quality)** you eat and **when (time)** you eat.

Starting with the "how" is intentional because it is more realistic to first of all control the quantity of what you eat and then make continuous progress from there.

- "How" refers to the **portion** of food: your waist line would definitely reveal the portion of food you eat. To cut down your portion, try using smaller bowls or flat plates. This would help keep it in check.

- "What" refers to the **proportion of nutritional content**: having a good enough combination of the different nutritional classes (carbohydrates, protein, fats, fiber, minerals, vitamins and water) in your meal, helps in keeping you healthy. Your diet should be balanced at all times.

- "When" refers to the **time** of the day you eat: avoid being a night time nosher. The earlier you end your eating activities in a day, the faster the digestion process would be. This would leave you lighter, healthier and active.

In addition, water and sleep are essential. Insufficient drinking of water will obstruct the performance of the kidneys. This would prevent them from being able to flush wastes and toxins out of the body. One and half litres of water a day is sufficient. But if the weather is hot, more quantity should be drunk.

Taking a look at your urine before flushing, would help in determining whether or not you are drinking sufficient water. If your urine is light and clear then you are drinking sufficient water but if it is dark and unclear then you need to increase your water intake.

According to a scientific theory, getting insufficient sleep at night would cause you to opt for unhealthy meals. This causes you to eat around 566 calories more per day. Ladies, who sleep less than seven hours a night, have the likelihood of gaining 38% more weight than another person who sleeps more than seven hours a night. There is a high tendency of making healthy food choices when you decide on what your next meal would be, immediately after your current meal. Making spontaneous meal choices when you are already starving would cause you to settle for a detrimental meal.

Finally, eating takes time, create enough time to eat. You may finish your meal in three minutes, you have fed yourself but have you nourished yourself? When it is meal time, every other activity should be kept on hold. It is not about feeling guilty for missing something else by making time to eat but it is about realizing that you are worth sitting down and eating food.

Chapter 4 Do it yourself (DIY)

What you should not do is get obsessed with counting calories. What you should know, is the more processed your food is, the more its calorie content. The processing extent of your food can be controlled when you do the cooking yourself.

My brown haired fashion loving twelve year old niece Charity once engaged me in a discussion. She asked why there is such a thing as cooking. Not knowing the suitable response to provide, I asked her in return, do you like eating? I love eating, my niece responded. How then would you do the eating if the meal preparation does not take place? This question kept her thinking for a while.

My niece asked me that question because her mom has repeatedly said these words to her: *"you need to be with me in the kitchen so that you can also begin to learn how to cook"*. Of course this is a first class boring statement for a typical twelve year old. I shared my insight about cooking with her. I made her understand, that the statement made by her mom is not out of place. Reason being that a mother takes pride in seeing the replication of herself in her daughter as well as a father his son. It gives them an unexplainable joy.

Showing interest in cooking and learning how to cook only makes your mom less worried when she needs to spend more hours at work. She is assured that her little angel is able to stand in for her. This would give her no reason to stop by a fast food restaurant on her way home.

TRUTH ABOUT COOKING

The lack of colour in a meal highlights a limited range of nutrients. Cooking is not as stressful or complicated as you think, it is actually fun. Creativity and concentration are basically what is required. With creativity, something amazing is usually produced. A creative combination of herbs and spices would produce a yummy delicacy. The heart-warming feedbacks you receive from those who eat the meal you prepare would cause you to develop a genuine interest in cooking.

Choose to see the kitchen as a laboratory. A place where you go into, mix your creative ideas together and then come out with a mouth-watering discovery. When the meal does not turn out the way you intended it to turn out, do not beat yourself too hard. Just learn from it and then try again.

A served meal says a lot about the person who prepared it. You can to an extent tell how beautiful, colourful, happy, and generous the heart of the cook is. This can be determined from the presentation of the food, colour combination, the taste and quantity of the food. Ignite your creativity today, stay focused and keep showing the world that you have the best of hearts.

CHAPTER 5 MEAL SUGGESTIONS

I have put together some breakfast, lunch and dinner suggestions. These suggestions are flexible – they can be interchanged. You can have breakfast for dinner or lunch for breakfast. They can also be mixed with the regular staples in the area where you live.

BREAKFAST

1. Nutty-oat bar and ginger green tea

2. Green leafy vegetables and avocado

✓ Oats is known to support weight loss because of its fiber content.

✓ Green tea supports in weight loss. It contains polyphenols which function as powerful antioxidants.

✓ Ginger is high in gingerol, helps in proper digestion, acts as a remedy for nausea and has anti-inflammatory and antioxidant properties.

✓ Vegetables supply the body with potassium, folic acid and vitamins such as A, E and C. They help in keeping the internal systems in perfect condition.

✓ Avocado is highly nutritious and rich in healthy fats.

LUNCH

1. Potato medley

2. Rotmush palm oil sauce and white rice

✓ In an article written by a registered dietician, it is stated that all types of rice are packed with carbohydrates. The content of carbohydrate in three slices of bread is equivalent to the amount found in a cup of cooked rice, which is an average of 45 grams. A serving of rice providing 45 grams of carbohydrates will break down to about the same amount of sugar found in 11 teaspoons of sugar. This sugar ends up in the blood after being broken down.

✓ It is advised, that rice be paired with plenty of fiber-rich non-starchy vegetables, such as mushrooms, onions, red bell peppers, broccoli and cauliflower. As well as adequate amount of lean protein from chicken. Doing this boosts nutrient intake and lowers the impact on blood sugar.

DINNER

1. Vegken noodles

2. Grilled fish and salad

✓ The body utilizes protein for the building and repairing of tissues. Protein is necessary for developing muscles, bones and cartilage.

✓ Fish is packed with essential omega 3 fats and vitamin E which helps in reducing the risk of cardiovascular diseases and lowers the cholesterol level.

IN-BETWEEN MEALS AND SNACKS

Suggestions for in-between meals and snacks are; salad, stuffed-wraps, fresh fruits, boiled egg, nuts and seeds.

✓ Dried fruits contain more sugar and calories than fresh fruits. This is not because the production company added sugar to them (unless stated on the nutrient facts labels and ingredients) but because they are dehydrated. The dehydration process removes much water from the fruit. This removal of water removes some essential water based vitamins that can be obtained from fresh fruits.

✓ According to the United States Department of Agriculture's National Nutrient Database, one cup of raisins has over 434 calories and one cup of grapes has about 104 calories – same serving size but more pieces of dried fruits. One cup of raisins has over 80 grams of sugar while one cup of grapes has about 15 grams of sugar or less.

✓ Dried fruits are convenient and are not easily gotten tired of compared to fresh fruits – that is where the danger lies. You believe you are eating healthy whereas you are consuming more sugar than required. When you want to eat dried fruits please watch the quantity.

HEALTHY RELATIONSHIP WITH FOOD

Food is not the devil. There is no good or bad food, but your experience with food could be good or bad. There is a thing line between thinking carefully about what you eat and getting obsessed over it. Having a sense of what your body needs and eating mindfully eliminates the fear of eating too much and consequently gaining weight. Upholding a good relationship with food is not all about being a perfectionist but about eating moderate and clean.

As long as you keep it moderate and clean, you can eat what you want to eat. Over indulgence is the hindrance to a beautiful figure.

Chocolates are more a treat than a snack. They are not an abomination but should not be abused. If they are a tempting food for you, do not have them at home, so you would have to leave home to get a taste. For example, you really love chocolates, rather than having them sitting in your fridge screaming your name, you could go out for a chocolate at least once a week.

Balance out rather than make up. There is usually this instinct of wanting to make up for a food choice when you feel guilty. You make up for it either by being excessively restrictive at the next meal or working out for extra hours. Balancing out involves being less restrictive at a later meal even though you may have indulged at your previous meal.

Having a lighter meal after indulging, protects you from becoming excessively hungry as well as binging. You can slowly balance out over the week but not within the same day.

Chapter 6 Recipes and Procedures

Nutty-oat bar (six servings)

Ingredients

- Two medium glasses of oats

- ½ medium glass of milk

- Two table spoons of honey

- Two table spoons of creamy peanut butter

- Three tea spoons of sesame or coconut flakes

- Three pinches of salt

Procedure

1. Do not preheat oven.

2. Mixture should be done with anything other than a mixer.

3. In a bowl slightly mix oats, milk and salt.

4. Add honey, peanut butter and sesame or coconut flakes and mix thoroughly. Set aside.

5. Lay an aluminium sheet on your oven tray, grease it with a little bit of groundnut oil or butter then turn out mixture on the tray. Form the mixture into a shape that you want but a square or a rectangle is easier to achieve. This can be done either with hand or a table spoon.

6. Sprinkle sesame or coconut flakes on top of your formed shape then slide tray into the oven.

7. Bake for 40 minutes at 170°C or until brown.

8. Slice as desired.

Note: If you would love a more crunchy feeling, then use crunchy instead of creamy peanut butter.

GINGER-GREEN TEA (ONE SERVING)

INGREDIENTS

- Hot water

- Ginger (moderate portion)

- A bag of green tea

PROCEDURE

1. Boil water

2. Slice ginger into a tea cup, add hot water and allow sitting for two minutes.

3. Put in green tea bag and allow sitting for one minute.

4. Serve with ginger slices still in tea cup and without the green tea bag.

POTATO MEDLEY (ONE SERVING)

INGREDIENTS

- 3 medium sized Irish potatoes

- 1½ table spoon ground nut oil

- ½ onion bulb

- 1 garlic clove

- ¼ red bell pepper

- 1 medium sized carrot

- 2 chicken sausage sticks

- 2 peperoni sticks

- Salt, curry, thyme, and pepper to taste.

- Any cooking seasoning of your choice.

PROCEDURE

1. Dice and boil potatoes for 7 minutes, turn it into a sieve and set aside.

2. Dice and heat up carrot in the microwave for one minute.

3. Pour ground nut oil into a frying pan; add diced sausages, garlic and onions. Fry until

sausages begin to turn brown. Stir continuously and turn out fried sausages into a bowl, leaving the oil in the pan.

4. In the pan add the already boiled potatoes and spread them out, leaving none over the other.

5. As potatoes begin to turn gold, add curry, thyme, pepper, salt and cooking seasoning. Fry until potato is completely tender.

6. Add already fried sausage, heated up carrot and diced red bell pepper. Stir properly and turn off heat.

7. Serve and top it up with two peperoni sticks.

Note: You can make use of any sausage type.

ROTMUSH PALM OIL SAUCE AND WHITE RICE (FOUR SERVINGS)

INGREDIENTS

- 500g rice

- 150g mushrooms

- 150g palm oil

- 400g spinach

- 3 medium sized carrots

- 2 medium sized onions

- Salt and pepper to taste

- Any cooking seasoning and protein of your choice

PROCEDURE

1. Boil rice and carrot until soft. Set aside.

2. Boil chicken till tender. Set aside.

3. In another pot pour in palm oil, allow it to heat up for 30 seconds and add chopped onions. Keep stirring as you allow frying for two minutes.

4. Add mushrooms, chicken, cooking seasoning, salt and pepper. Allow to cook for six minutes.

5. Add spinach, cook for three minutes, stir properly and taste for salt.

6. Serve.

Note: If it turns out too thick, add some water.

VEGKEN NOODLES/ GRILLED FISH AND SALAD

Under this category, there are no strict guidelines. You can be as creative as you want. You can make use of any form of pasta, green vegetable and protein. Prepare it to your taste.

Prepare your salad just the way you love it. But here is a tip: gather the vegetables you would like to make use of and nicely slice them. Turn the nicely sliced vegetables into a bowl and add: a little bit of salt, vinegar, black pepper, boiled and diced chicken breast, sliced parsley and one diced apple. The quantity of each item would vary in accordance with the quantity of salad you intending preparing. With these ingredients in your salad, there would be no need for mayonnaise. But if you must make use of mayonnaise, be moderate about it. A table spoon of mayonnaise contains 94 calories. Buy any fish of your choice and grill it the way it best appeals to you.

Chapter 7 Welcome on Board

You are beautiful and no one should convince you otherwise. You do not need to wait for someone to recite those words to you before you believe it. That is who and what you are, beautiful. Say it to yourself as many times a possible until you are convinced that you are beautiful.

You are the sailor of your ship, when you come across anyone who tries to ridicule, judge or mock you because of your looks, please sail on! Those who believe that you worth much more than your looks and you are a work in progress are welcome on board.

Stay motivated and patient until you reach your goal.

OTHER BOOKS BY IRUOMA AWO

Discover New Perspectives

Empathy and Affection

What Next after Graduation?

Unschlagbarer Entdeckungen

www.ingramcontent.com/pod-product-compliance
Lightning Source LLC
Chambersburg PA
CBHW060820260726
48660CB00003B/1016